Quit Smoking

Colouring Journal
6 month Tracker

This Journal Belongs to:

Name: _______________________

Tel: _______________________

Email: _______________________

My Future Plans

For Myself

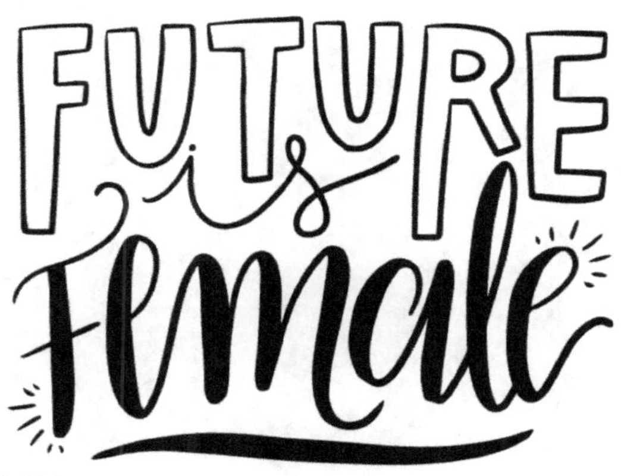

For Family

Top 3 Goals

6 MONTH Plan

START DATE:

Personal life

Work life

Kick the habit month 1

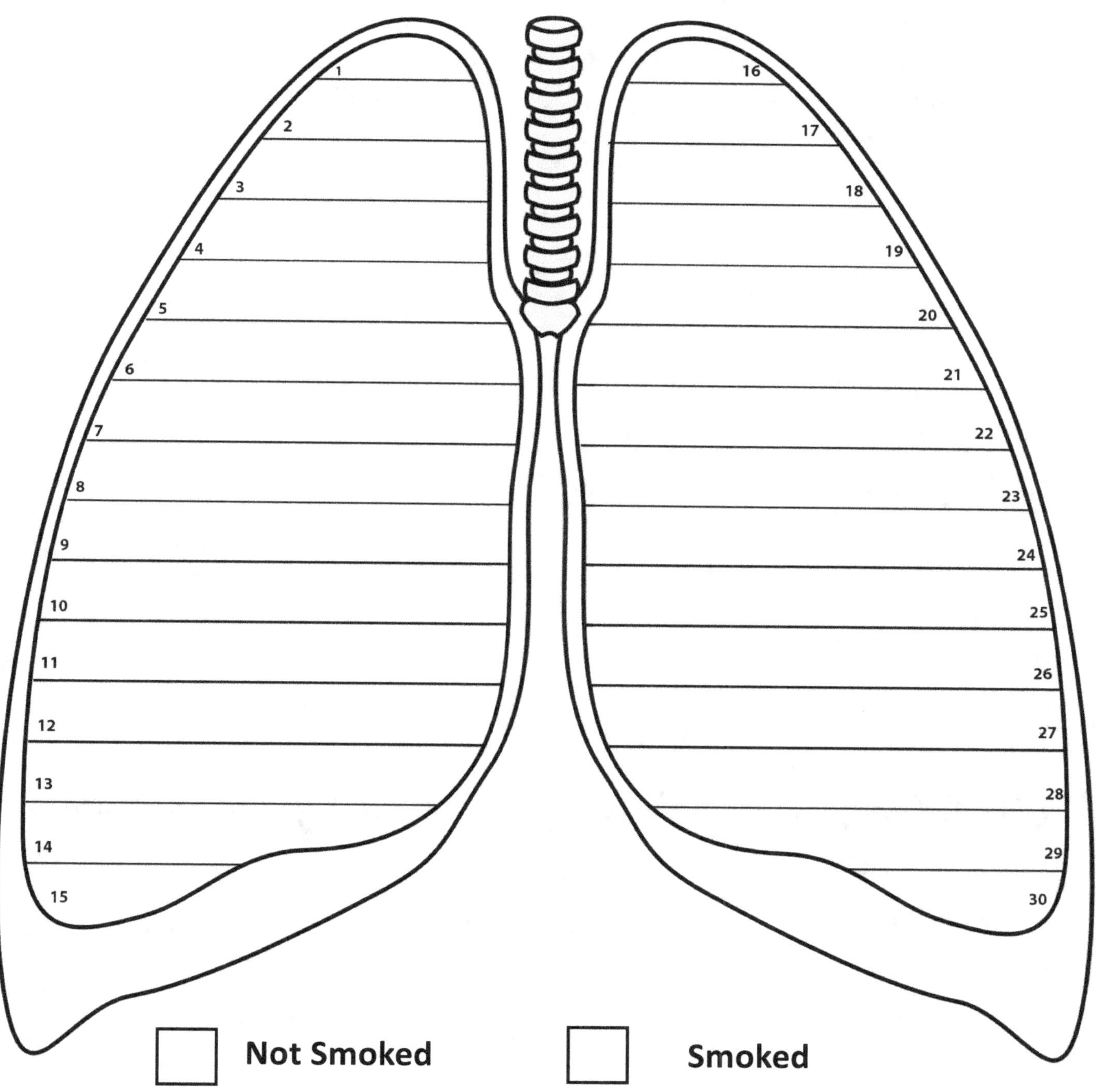

"It is in your moments of decision that your destiny is shaped. "- Tony Robbins

Week

MONTH:

WEEK:

WEEKLY WINS

WORK IN PROGRESS

One Step at a time, One Day at a time

MY GOALS

FAMILY GOALS

CAREER GOALS

Today

MON

TUE

WED

THU

Today

FRI

SAT

SUN

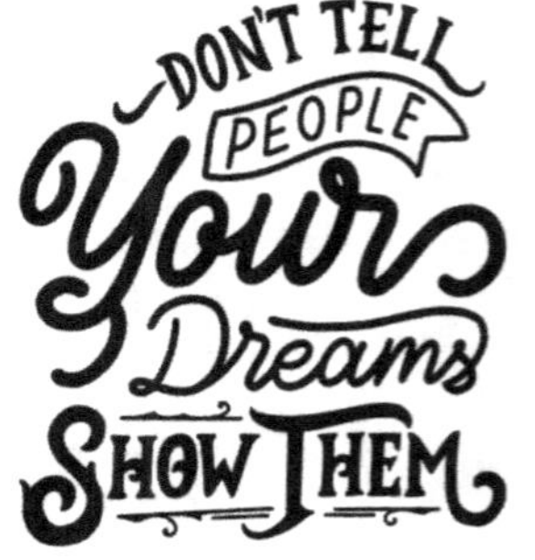

Week

MONTH: WEEK:

WEEKLY WINS	WORK IN PROGRESS

One Step at a time, One Day at a time

MY GOALS	FAMILY GOALS	CAREER GOALS

Today

MON

TUE

WED

THU

Today

FRI

SAT

SUN

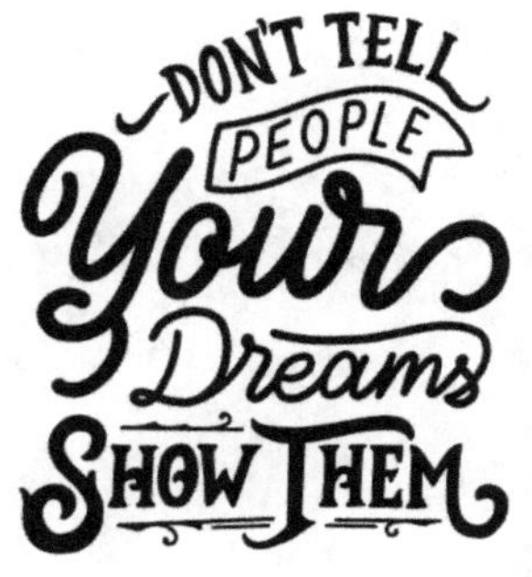

Week

MONTH:

WEEK:

WEEKLY WINS

WORK IN PROGRESS

One Step at a time, One Day at a time

MY GOALS

FAMILY GOALS

CAREER GOALS

Today

MON

TUE

WED

THU

Today

FRI

SAT

SUN

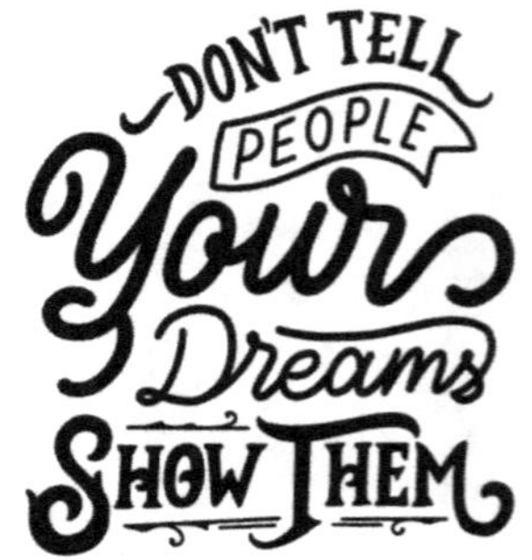

Week

MONTH:

WEEK:

WEEKLY WINS	WORK IN PROGRESS

One Step at a time, One Day at a time

MY GOALS	FAMILY GOALS	CAREER GOALS

Today

MON

TUE

WED

THU

Today

FRI

SAT

SUN

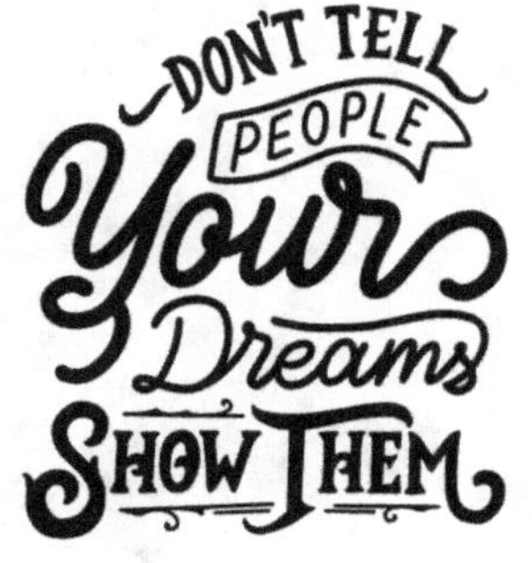

Week

MONTH: WEEK:

WEEKLY WINS	WORK IN PROGRESS

One Step at a time, One Day at a time

MY GOALS	FAMILY GOALS	CAREER GOALS

Today

MON

TUE

WED

THU

Today

FRI

SAT

SUN

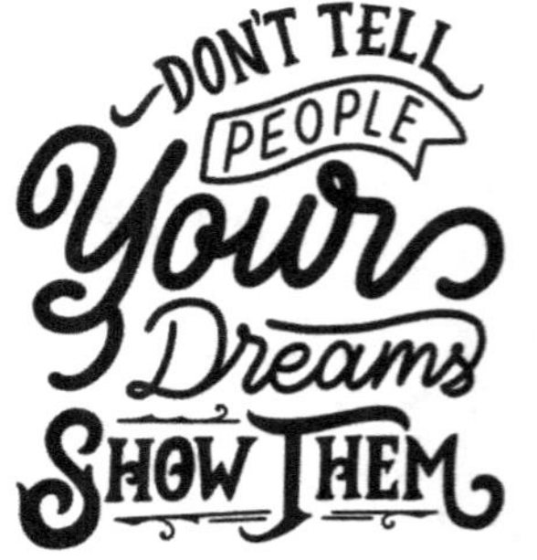

How I Felt

Combat Techniques

Reflections of this month

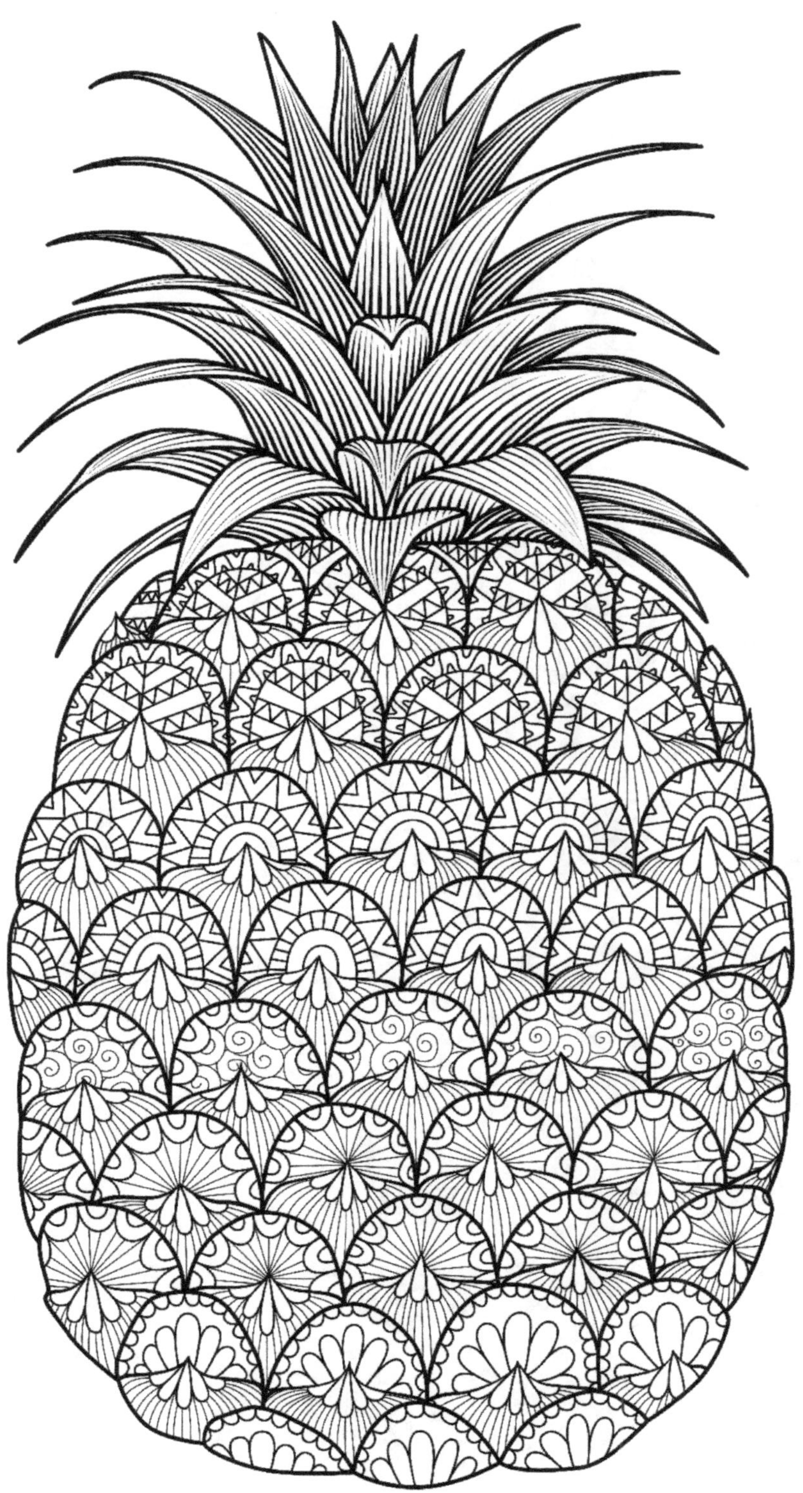

For the first few days after you quit smoking, spend as much free time as you can in public places where smoking is not allowed. (Libraries, malls, museums, theaters, restaurants without bars, and churches are most often smoke-free.)

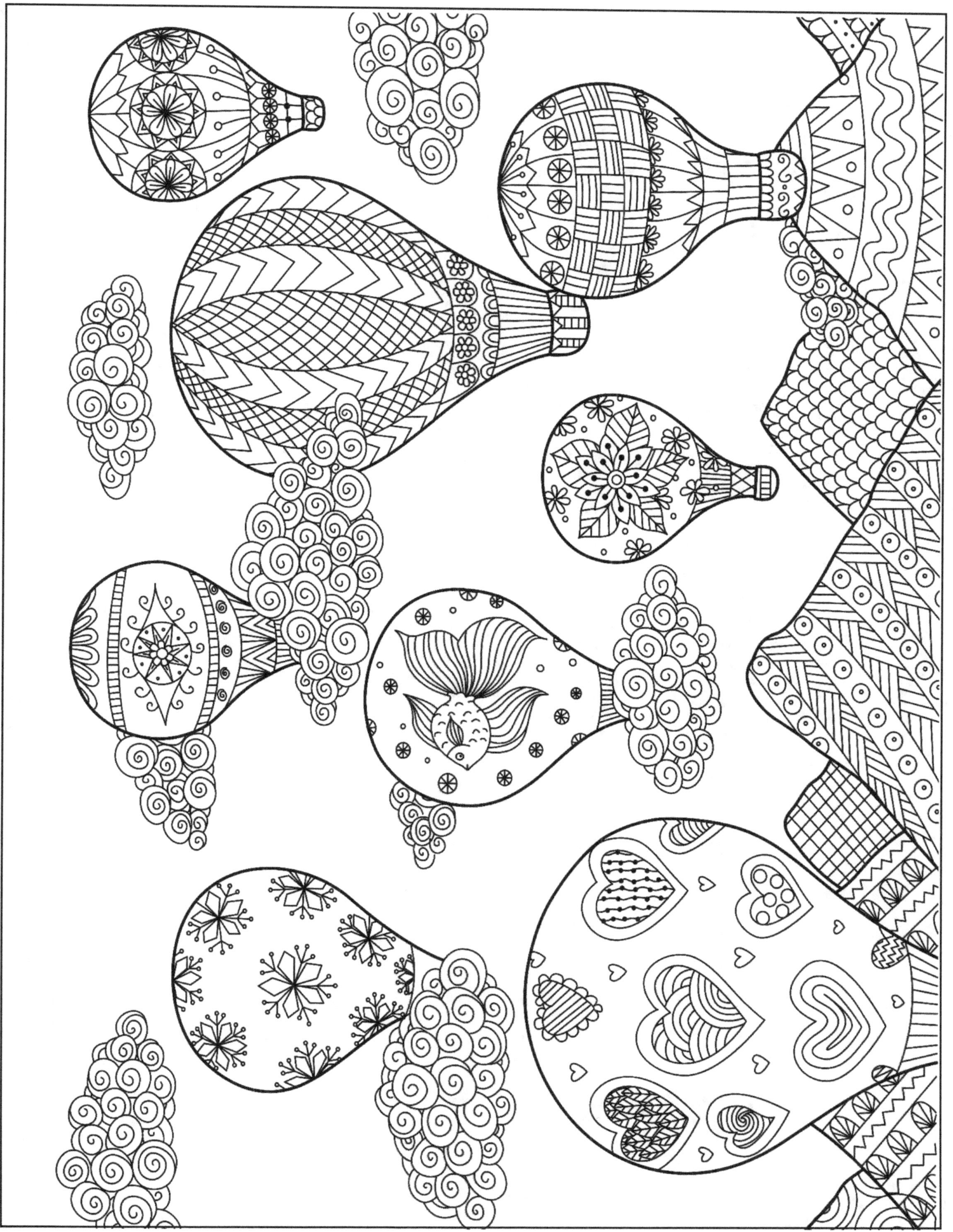

Kick the habit month 2

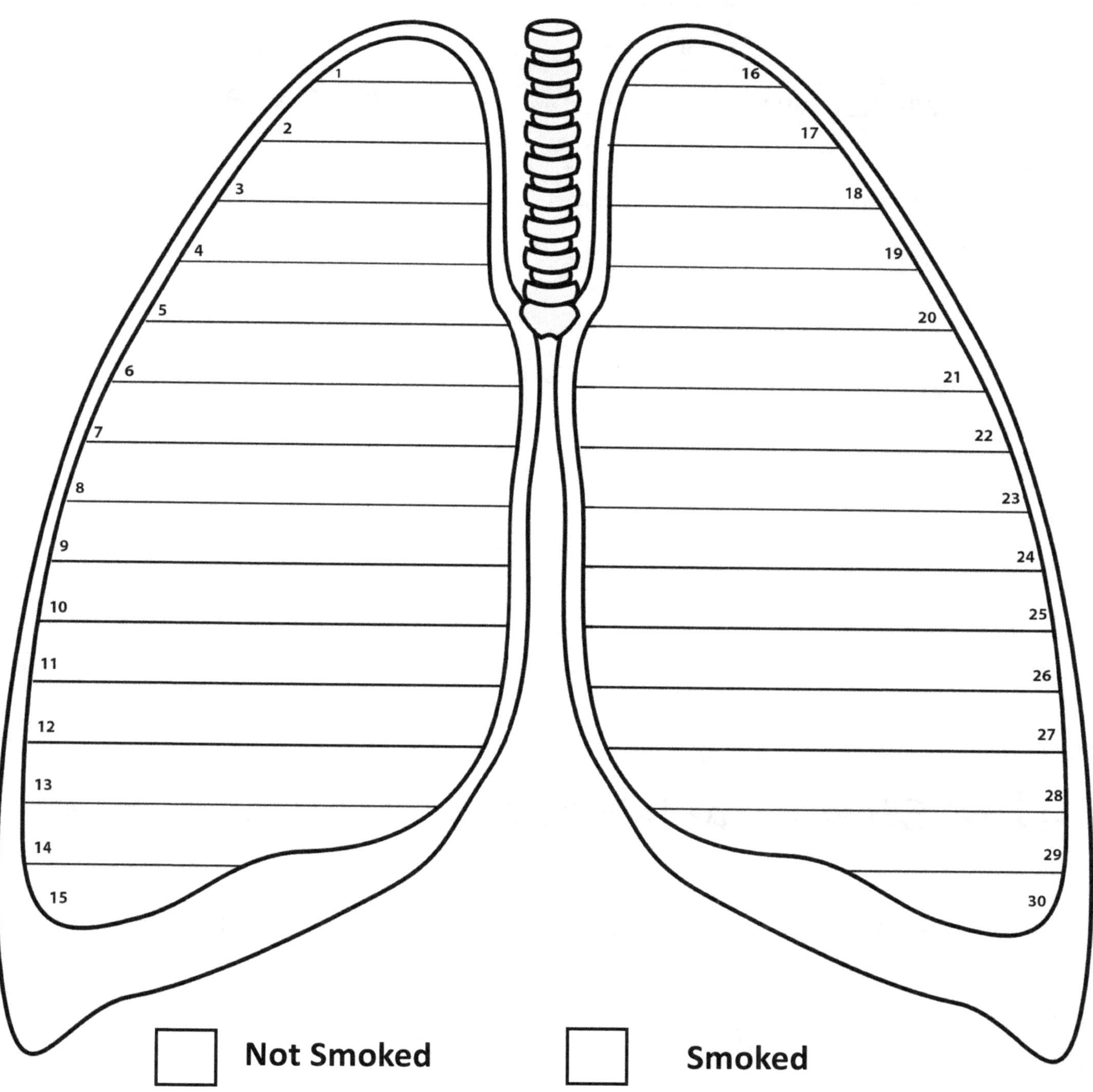

"The secret of getting ahead is getting started." - Mark Twain

Week

MONTH: WEEK:

WEEKLY WINS	WORK IN PROGRESS

One Step at a time, One Day at a time

MY GOALS	FAMILY GOALS	CAREER GOALS

Today

MON

TUE

WED

THU

Today

FRI

SAT

SUN

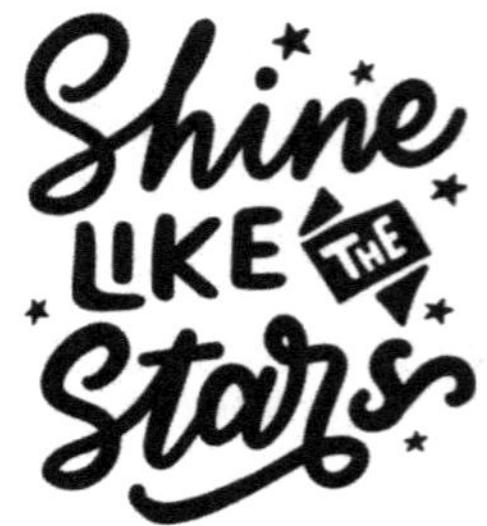

Week

MONTH: WEEK:

WEEKLY WINS	WORK IN PROGRESS

One Step at a time, One Day at a time

MY GOALS	FAMILY GOALS	CAREER GOALS

Today

MON

TUE

WED

THU

Today

FRI

SAT

SUN

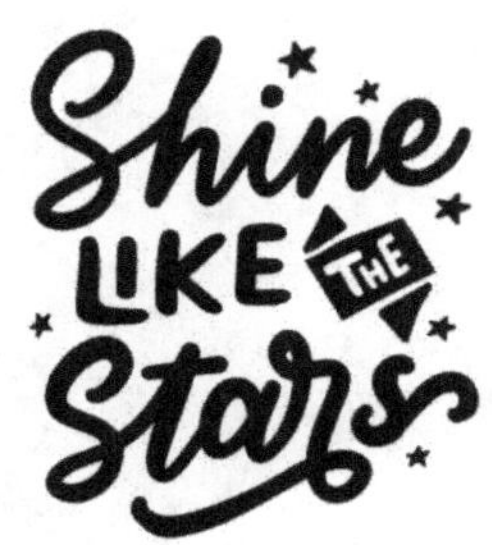

Week

MONTH:

WEEK:

WEEKLY WINS

WORK IN PROGRESS

One Step at a time, One Day at a time

MY GOALS

FAMILY GOALS

CAREER GOALS

Today

MON

TUE

WED

THU

Today

FRI

SAT

SUN

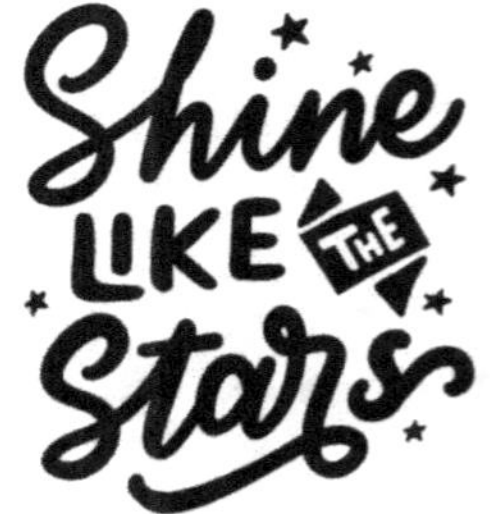

Week

MONTH:

WEEK:

WEEKLY WINS	WORK IN PROGRESS

One Step at a time, One Day at a time

MY GOALS	FAMILY GOALS	CAREER GOALS

Today

MON

TUE

WED

THU

Today

FRI

SAT

SUN

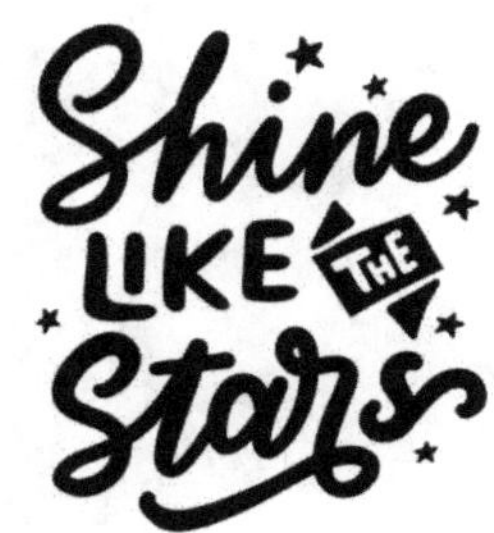

Week

MONTH:

WEEK:

WEEKLY WINS

WORK IN PROGRESS

One Step at a time, One Day at a time

MY GOALS

FAMILY GOALS

CAREER GOALS

Today

MON

TUE

WED

THU

Today

FRI

SAT

SUN

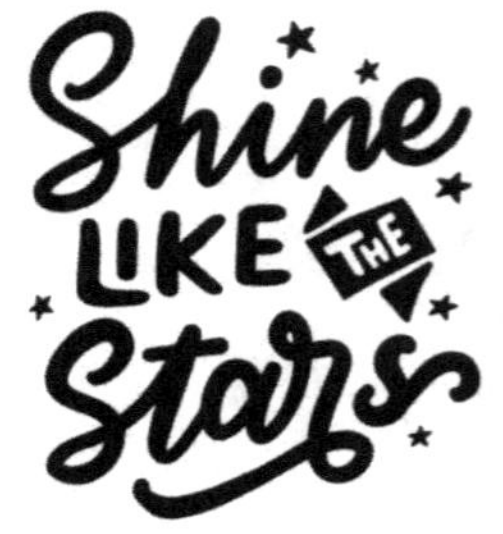

How I Felt

Combat Techniques

Reflections of this month

Color the stress away...

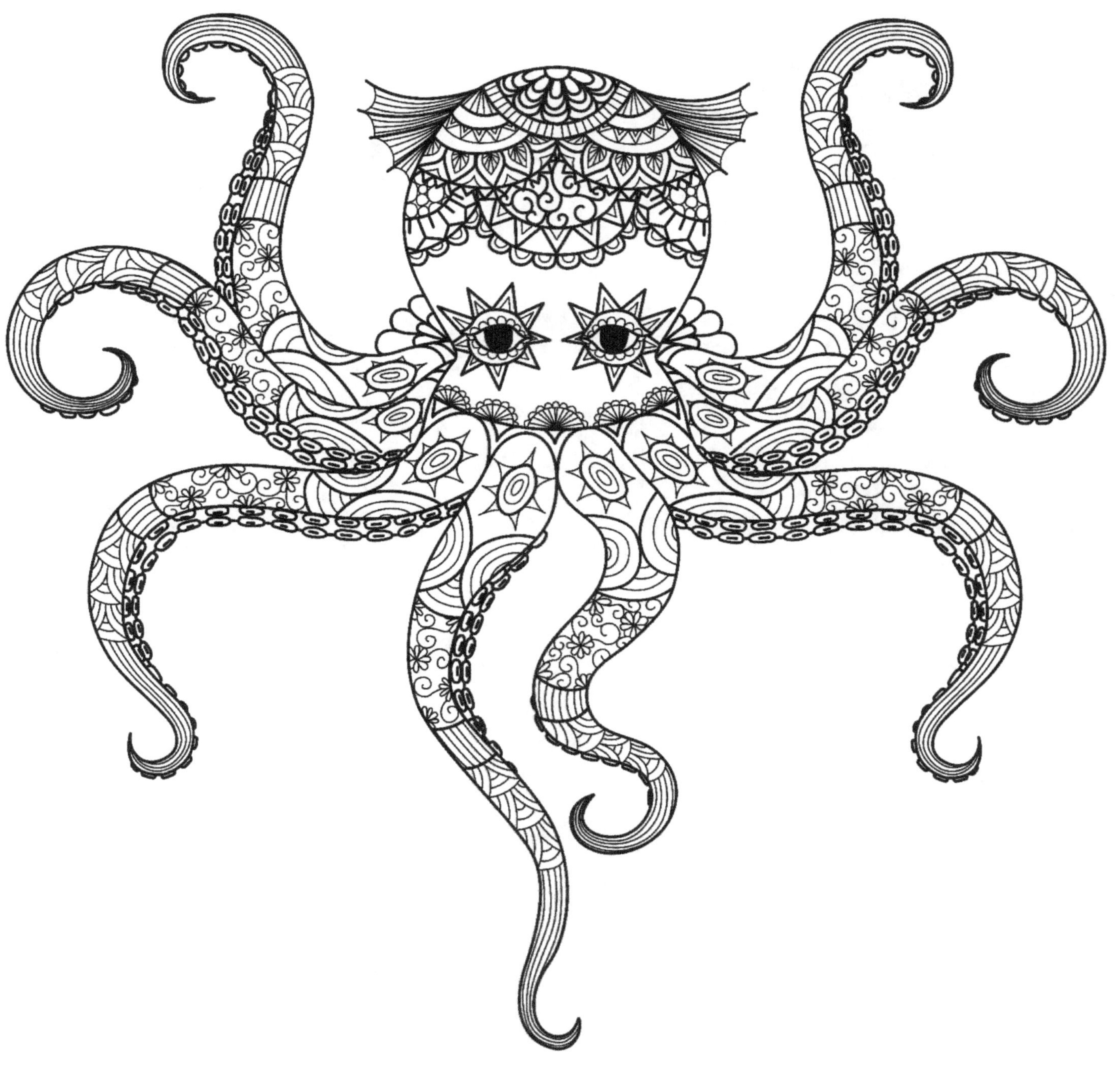

Take extra care of yourself. Drink water, eat well, and get enough sleep. This could help you have the energy you might need to handle extra stress.

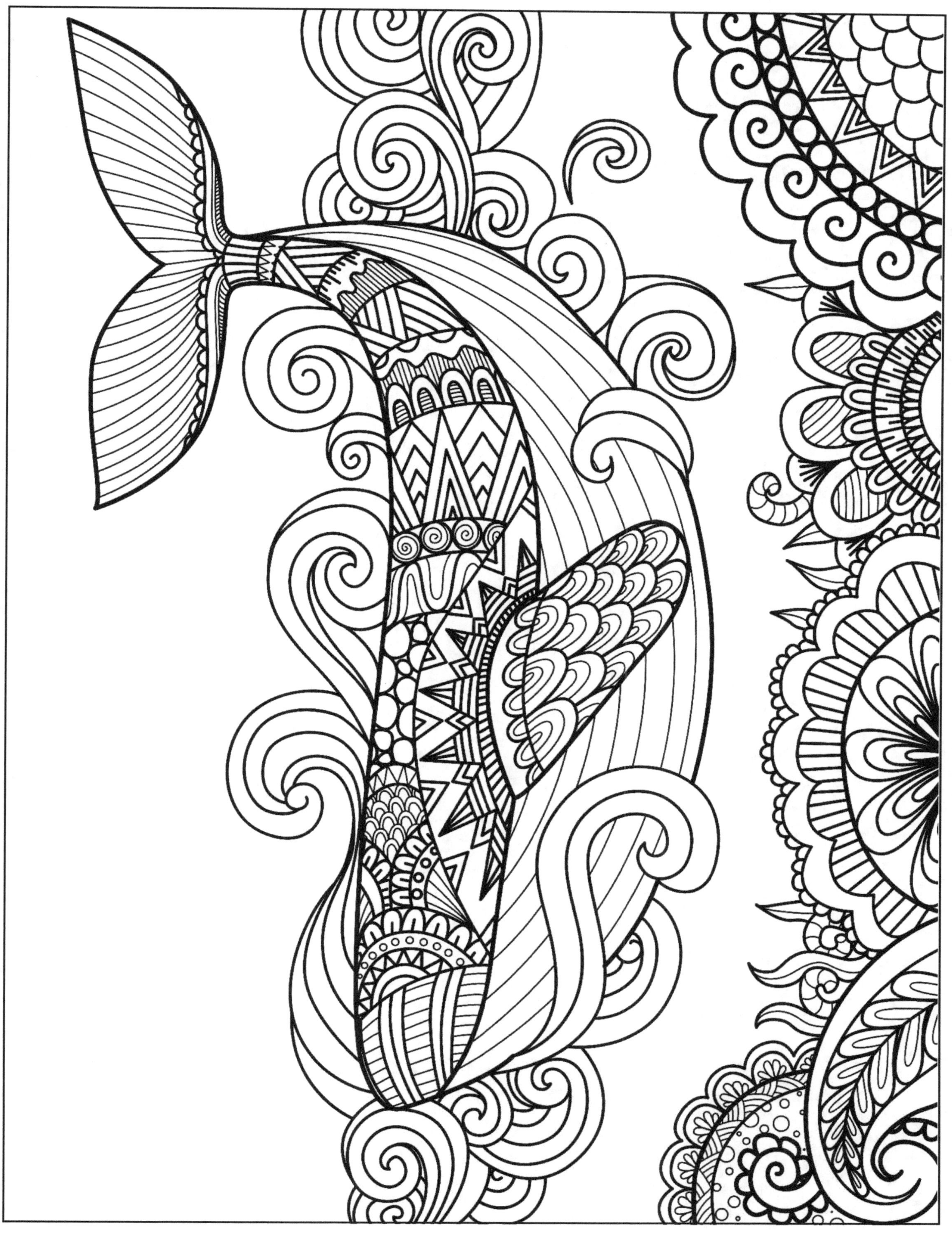

Kick the habit month 3

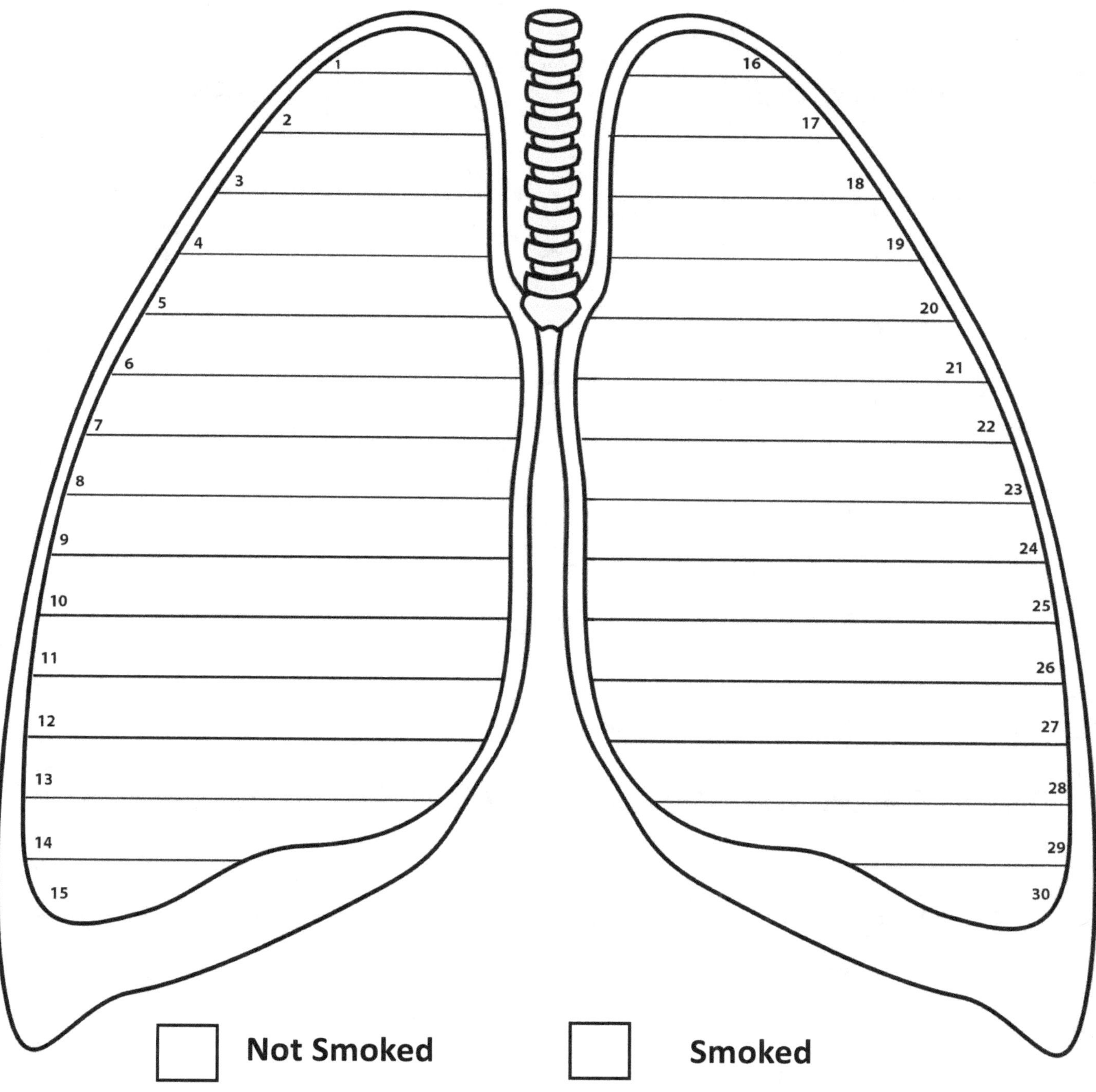

☐ **Not Smoked**   ☐ **Smoked**

"Believe you can and you're halfway there." - Theodore
Roosevelt

Week

MONTH:

WEEK:

WEEKLY WINS	WORK IN PROGRESS

One Step at a time, One Day at a time

MY GOALS	FAMILY GOALS	CAREER GOALS

Today

MON

TUE

WED

THU

Today

FRI

SAT

SUN

You are awesome

Week

MONTH:

WEEK:

WEEKLY WINS	WORK IN PROGRESS

One Step at a time, One Day at a time

MY GOALS	FAMILY GOALS	CAREER GOALS

Today

MON

TUE

WED

THU

Today

FRI

SAT

SUN

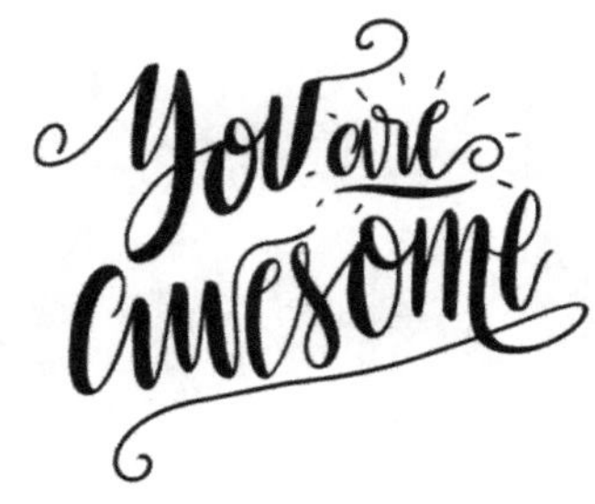

Week

MONTH:

WEEK:

WEEKLY WINS

WORK IN PROGRESS

One Step at a time, One Day at a time

MY GOALS

FAMILY GOALS

CAREER GOALS

Today

MON

TUE

WED

THU

Today

FRI

SAT

SUN

Week

MONTH: WEEK:

WEEKLY WINS	WORK IN PROGRESS

One Step at a time, One Day at a time

MY GOALS	FAMILY GOALS	CAREER GOALS

Today

MON

TUE

WED

THU

Today

FRI

SAT

SUN

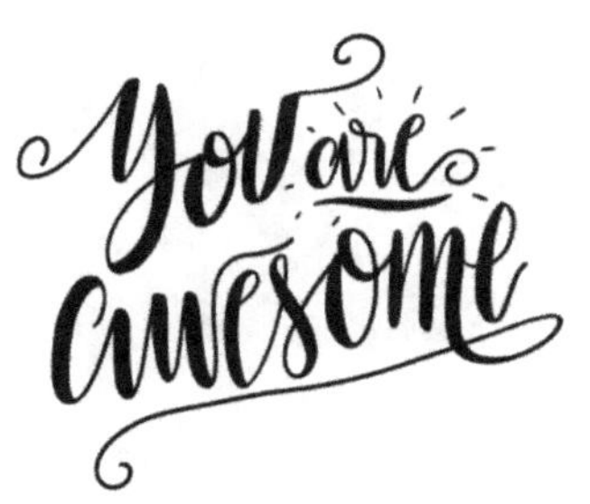

Week

MONTH:

WEEK:

WEEKLY WINS	WORK IN PROGRESS

One Step at a time, One Day at a time

MY GOALS	FAMILY GOALS	CAREER GOALS

Today

MON

TUE

WED

THU

Today

FRI

SAT

SUN

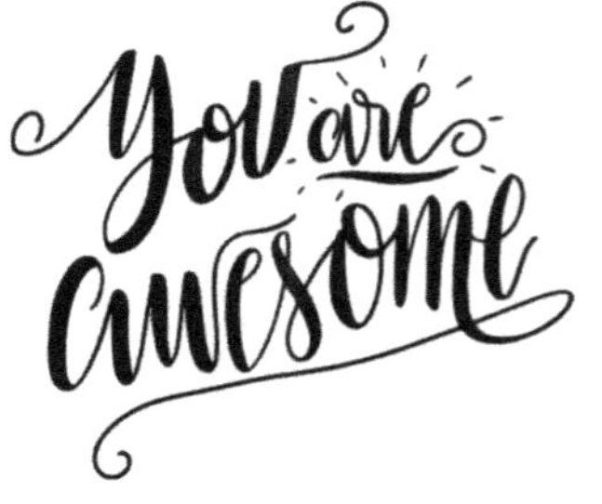

How I Felt

Combat Techniques

Reflections of this month

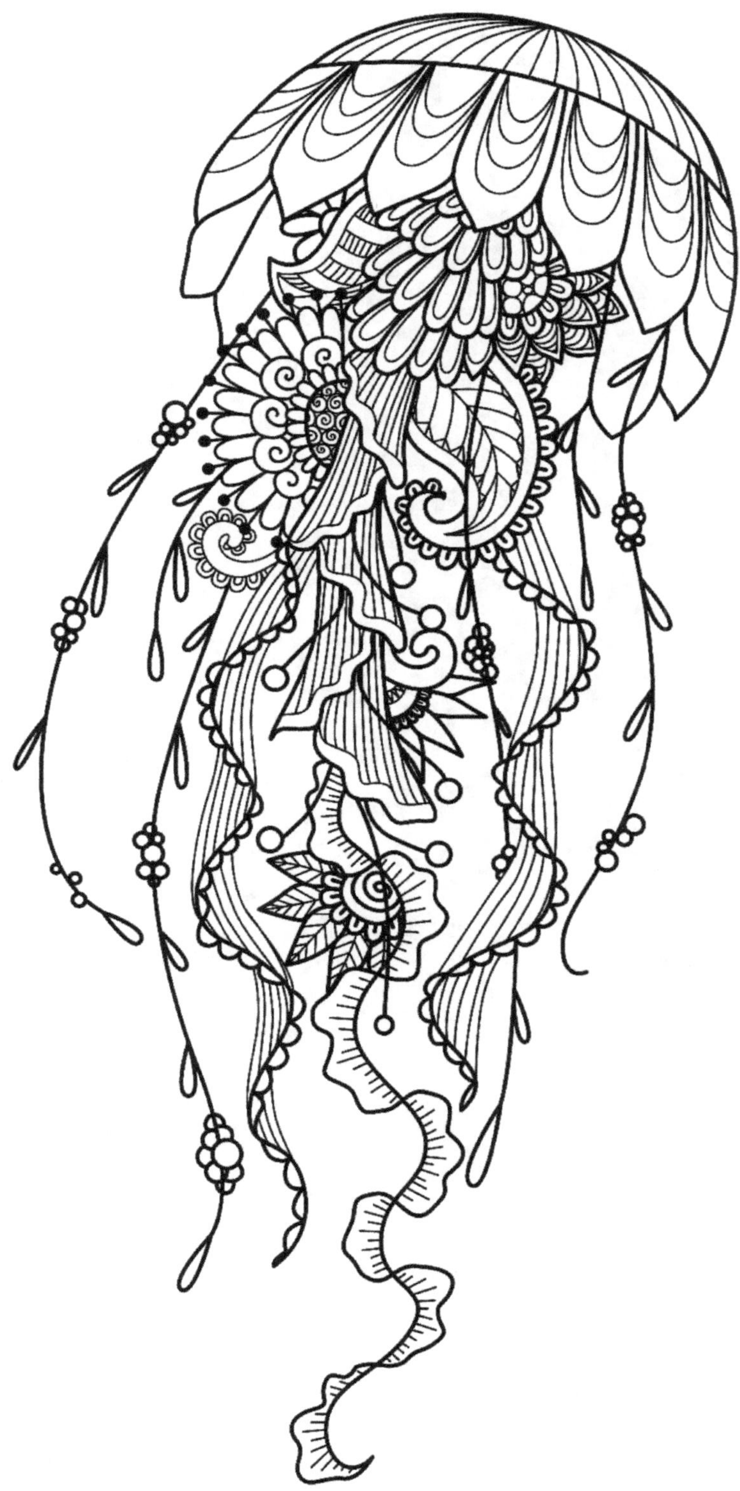

Don't drink alcohol, coffee, or any other drinks you link with smoking for at least a couple of months. Try something else instead – maybe different types of water, sports drinks, or 100% fruit juices. Try to choose drinks that are low- or no-calorie.

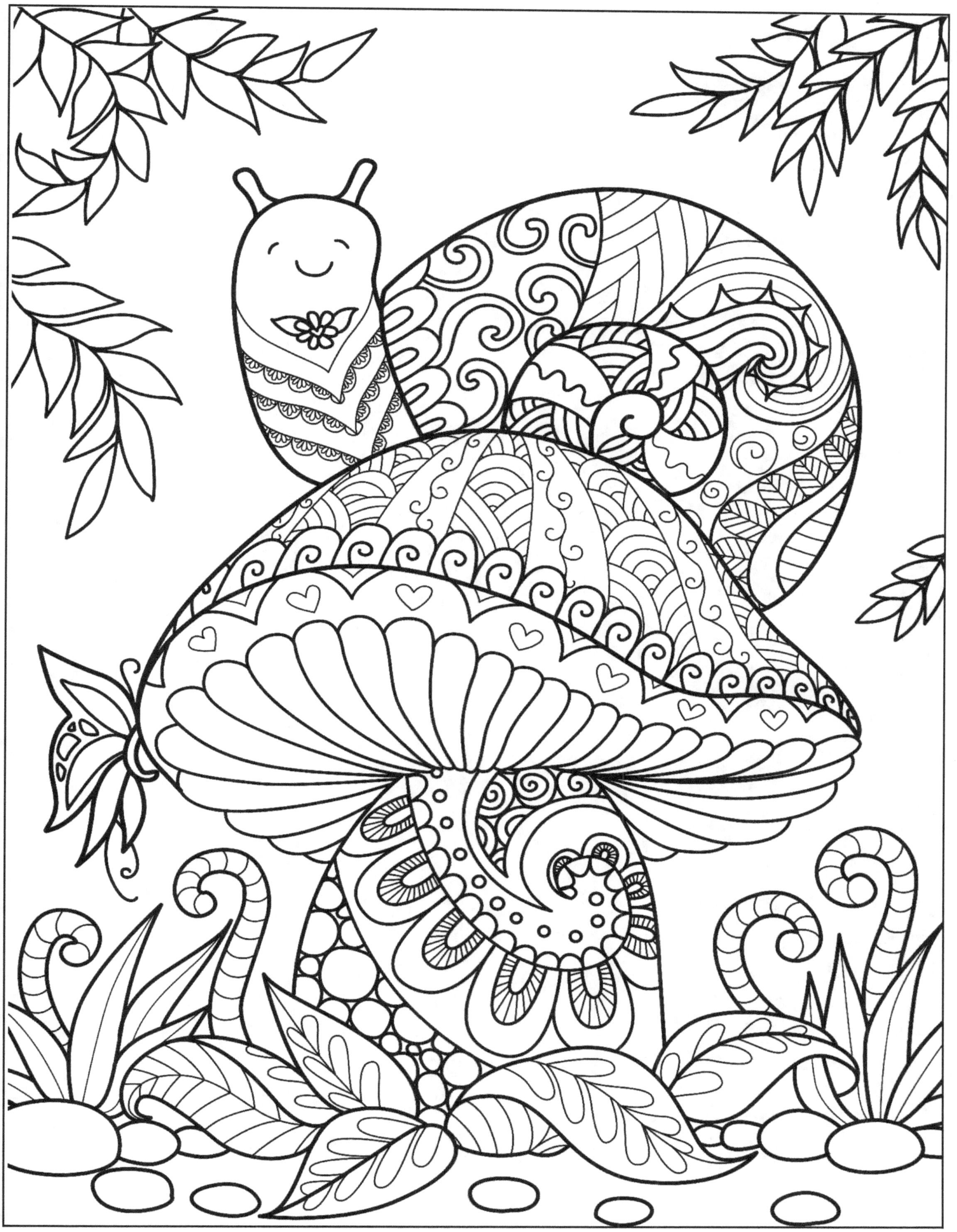

Kick the habit month 4

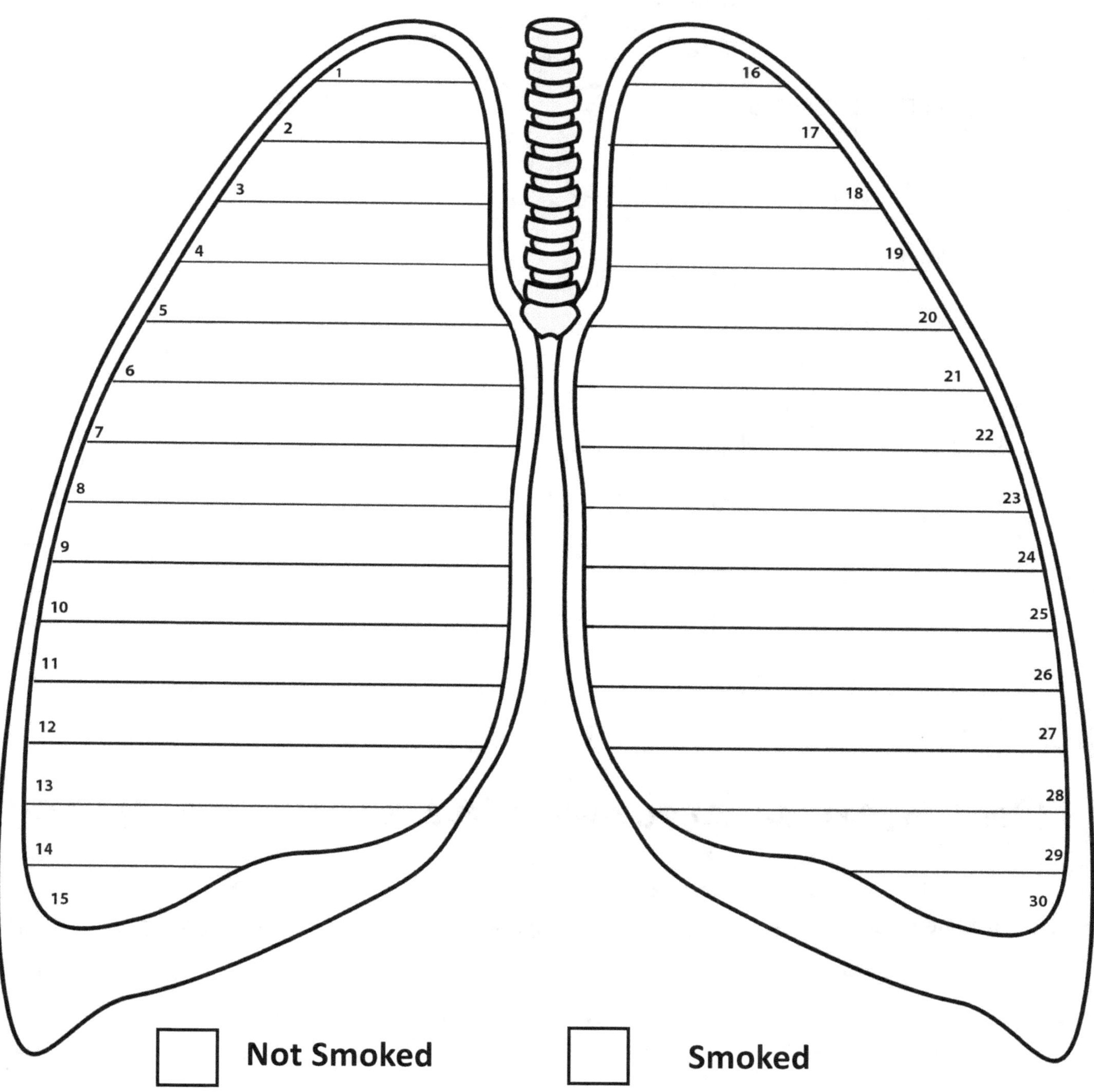

"Our strength grows out of our weakness." - Ralph Waldo Emerson

Week

MONTH:

WEEK:

WEEKLY WINS

WORK IN PROGRESS

One Step at a time, One Day at a time

MY GOALS

FAMILY GOALS

CAREER GOALS

Today

MON

TUE

WED

THU

Today

FRI

SAT

SUN

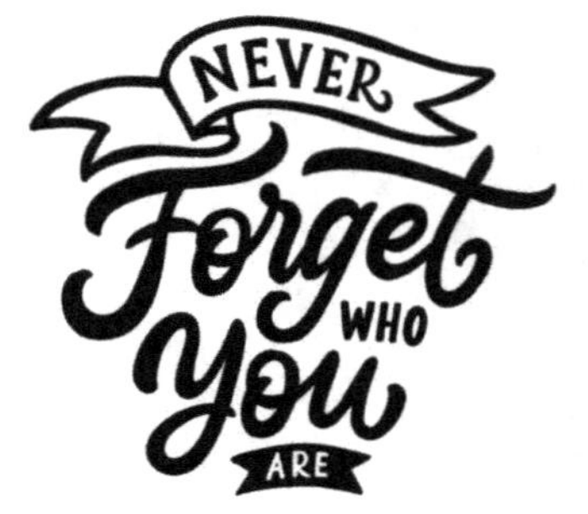

Week

MONTH:

WEEK:

WEEKLY WINS

WORK IN PROGRESS

One Step at a time, One Day at a time

MY GOALS

FAMILY GOALS

CAREER GOALS

Today

MON

TUE

WED

THU

Today

FRI

SAT

SUN

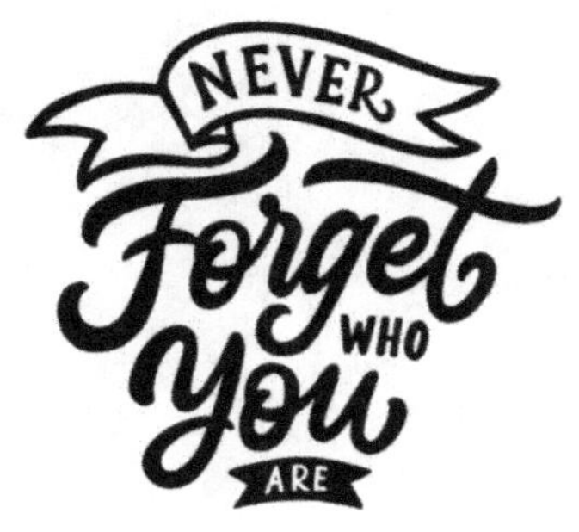

Week

MONTH:

WEEK:

WEEKLY WINS	WORK IN PROGRESS

One Step at a time, One Day at a time

MY GOALS	FAMILY GOALS	CAREER GOALS

Today

MON

TUE

WED

THU

Today

FRI

SAT

SUN

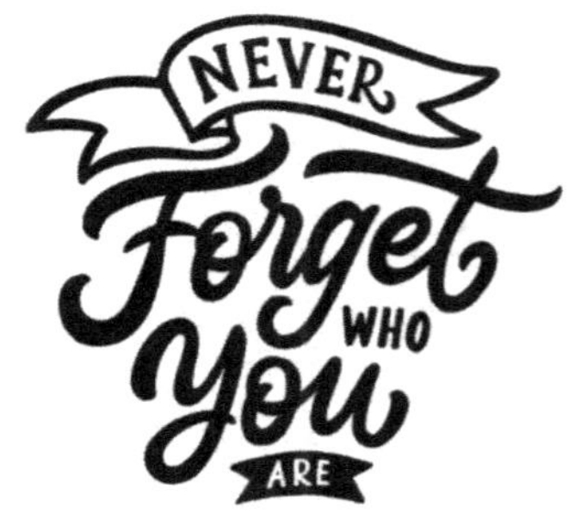

Week

MONTH:

WEEK:

WEEKLY WINS	WORK IN PROGRESS

One Step at a time, One Day at a time

MY GOALS	FAMILY GOALS	CAREER GOALS

Today

MON

TUE

WED

THU

Today

FRI

SAT

SUN

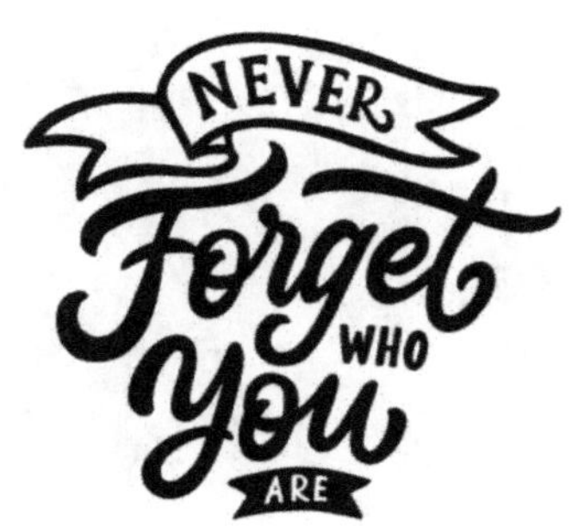

Week

MONTH:

WEEK:

WEEKLY WINS	WORK IN PROGRESS

One Step at a time, One Day at a time

MY GOALS	FAMILY GOALS	CAREER GOALS

Today

MON

TUE

WED

THU

Today

FRI

SAT

SUN

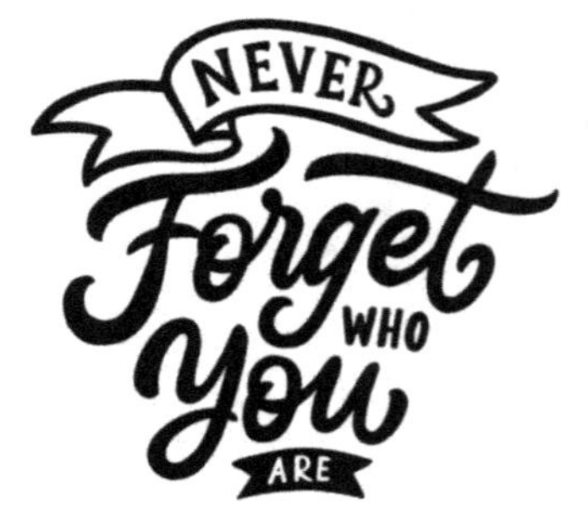

How I Felt

Combat Techniques

Reflections of this month

Color the stress away...

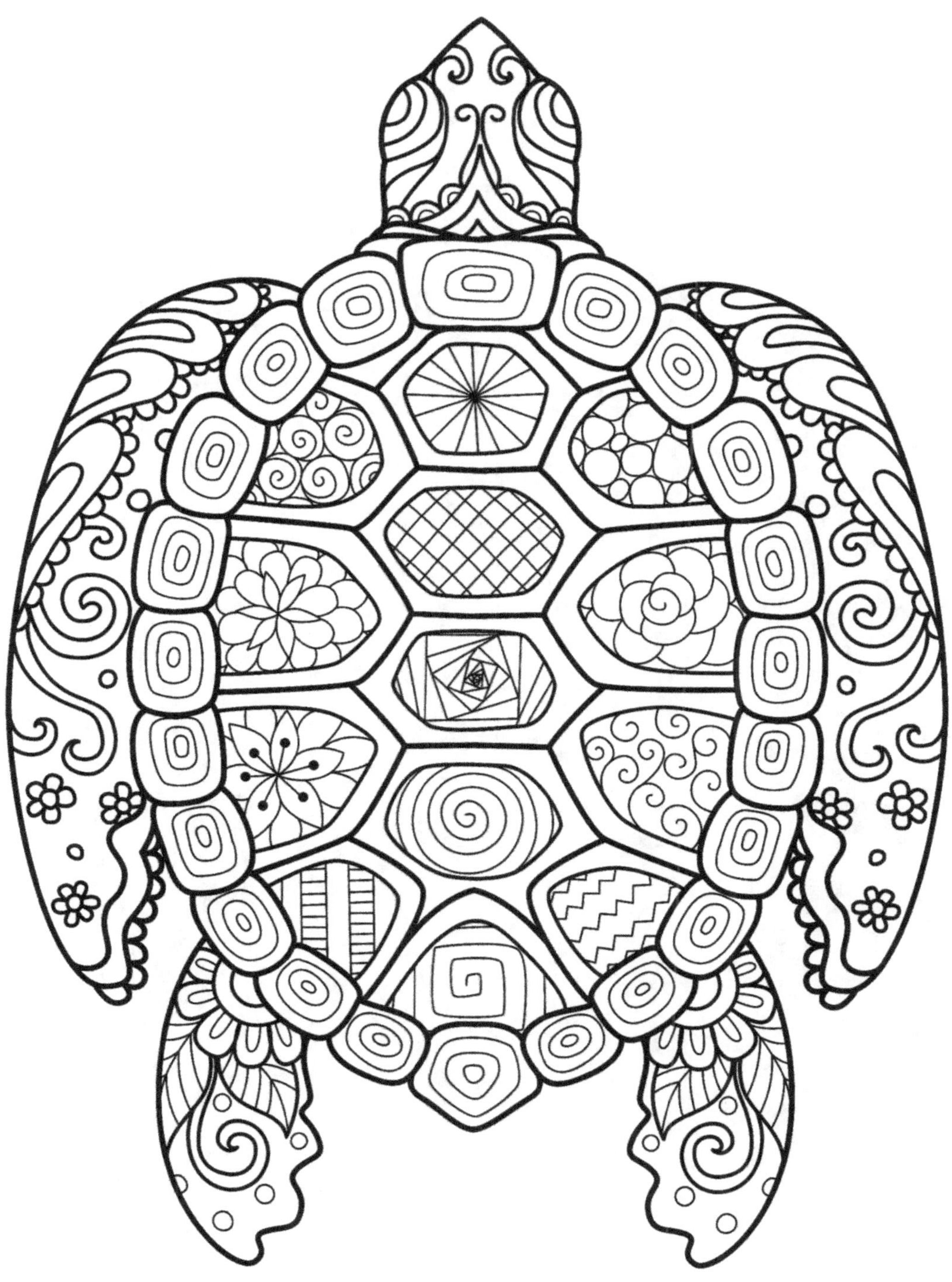

If you miss the feeling of having a cigarette in your hand, hold something else – a
pencil, a paper clip, a coin, or a marble, for example.

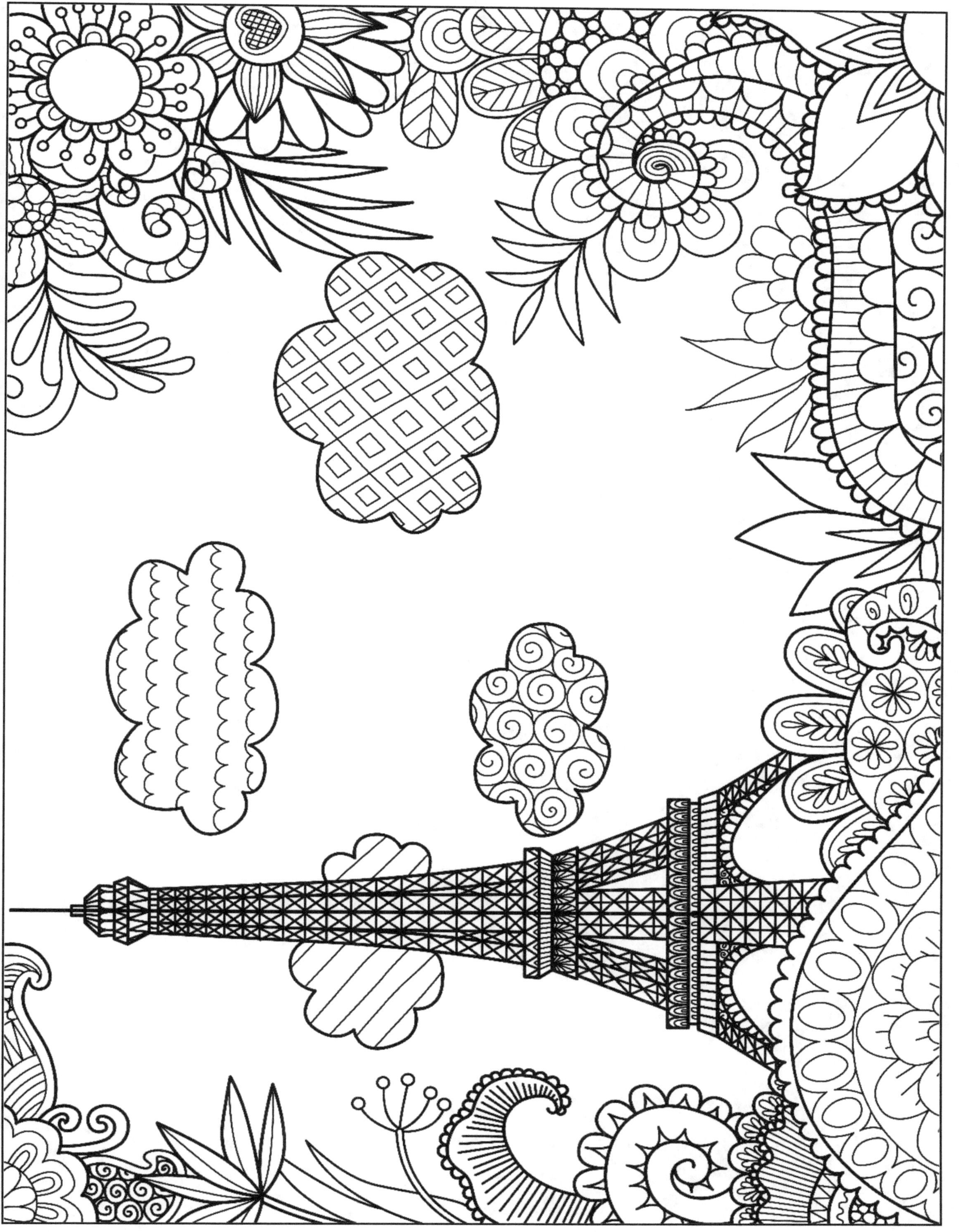

Kick the habit month 5

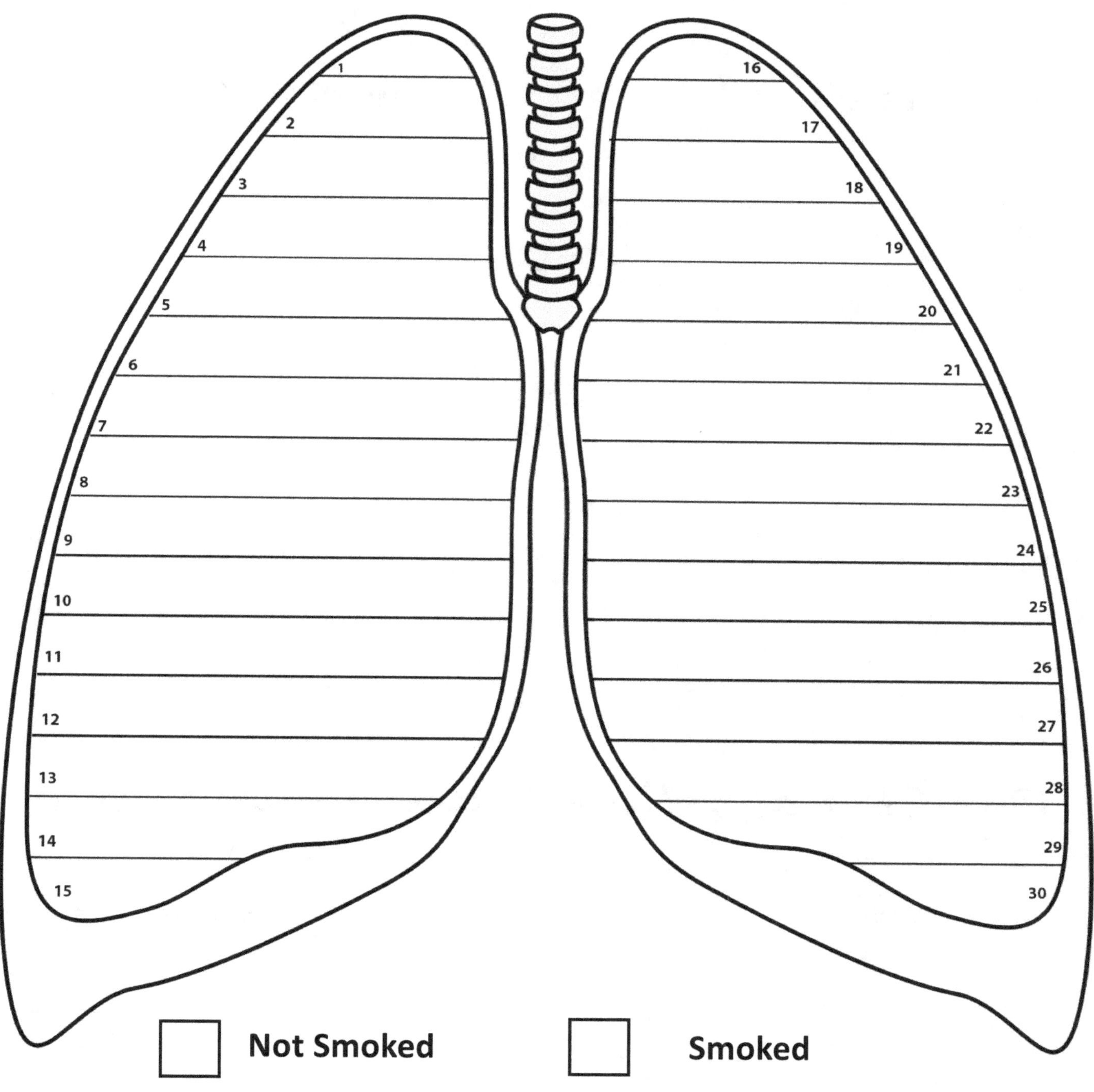

"We are what we repeatedly do. Excellence, then, is not an act, but a habit." - Aristotle

Week

MONTH:

WEEK:

WEEKLY WINS

WORK IN PROGRESS

One Step at a time, One Day at a time

MY GOALS

FAMILY GOALS

CAREER GOALS

Today

MON

TUE

WED

THU

Today

FRI

SAT

SUN

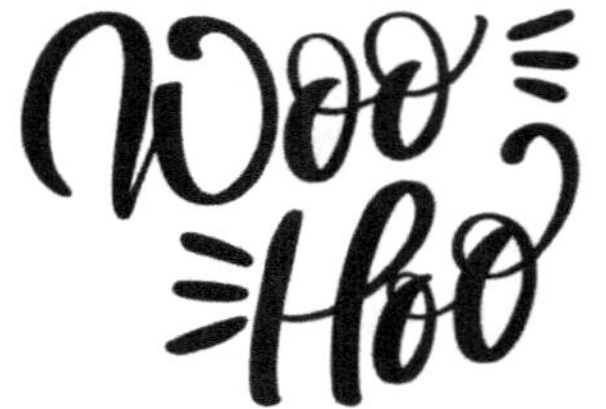

Week

MONTH: WEEK:

WEEKLY WINS	WORK IN PROGRESS

One Step at a time, One Day at a time

MY GOALS	FAMILY GOALS	CAREER GOALS

Today

DAILY
PLANNER

MON

TUE

WED

THU

Today

FRI

SAT

SUN

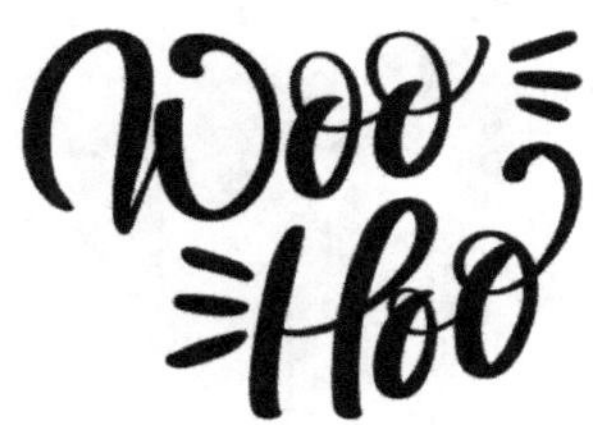

Week

MONTH:

WEEK:

WEEKLY WINS

WORK IN PROGRESS

One Step at a time, One Day at a time

MY GOALS

FAMILY GOALS

CAREER GOALS

Today

MON

TUE

WED

THU

Today

FRI

SAT

SUN

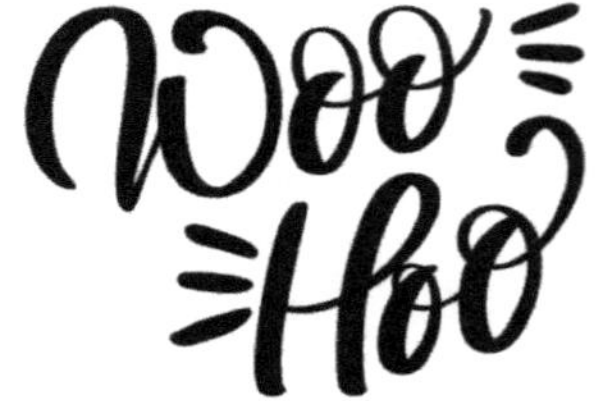

Week

MONTH:

WEEK:

WEEKLY WINS

WORK IN PROGRESS

One Step at a time, One Day at a time

MY GOALS

FAMILY GOALS

CAREER GOALS

Today

MON

TUE

WED

THU

Today

FRI

SAT

SUN

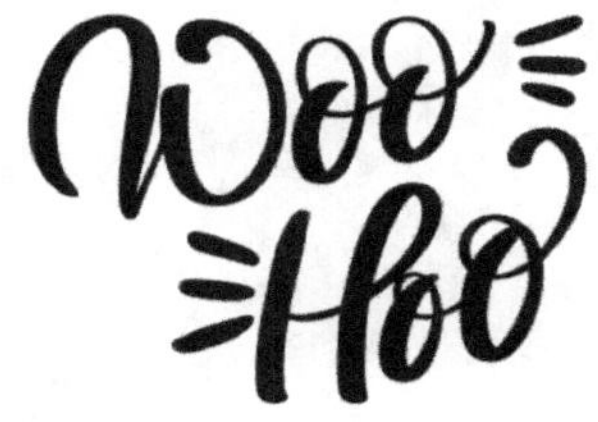

Week

MONTH:

WEEK:

WEEKLY WINS	WORK IN PROGRESS

One Step at a time, One Day at a time

MY GOALS	FAMILY GOALS	CAREER GOALS

Today

DAILY
PLANNER

MON

TUE

WED

THU

Today

FRI

SAT

SUN

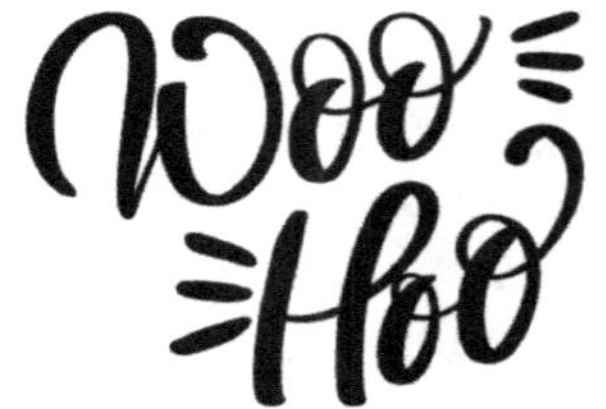

How I Felt

____

____

____

____

Combat Techniques

____

____

____

____

Reflections of this month

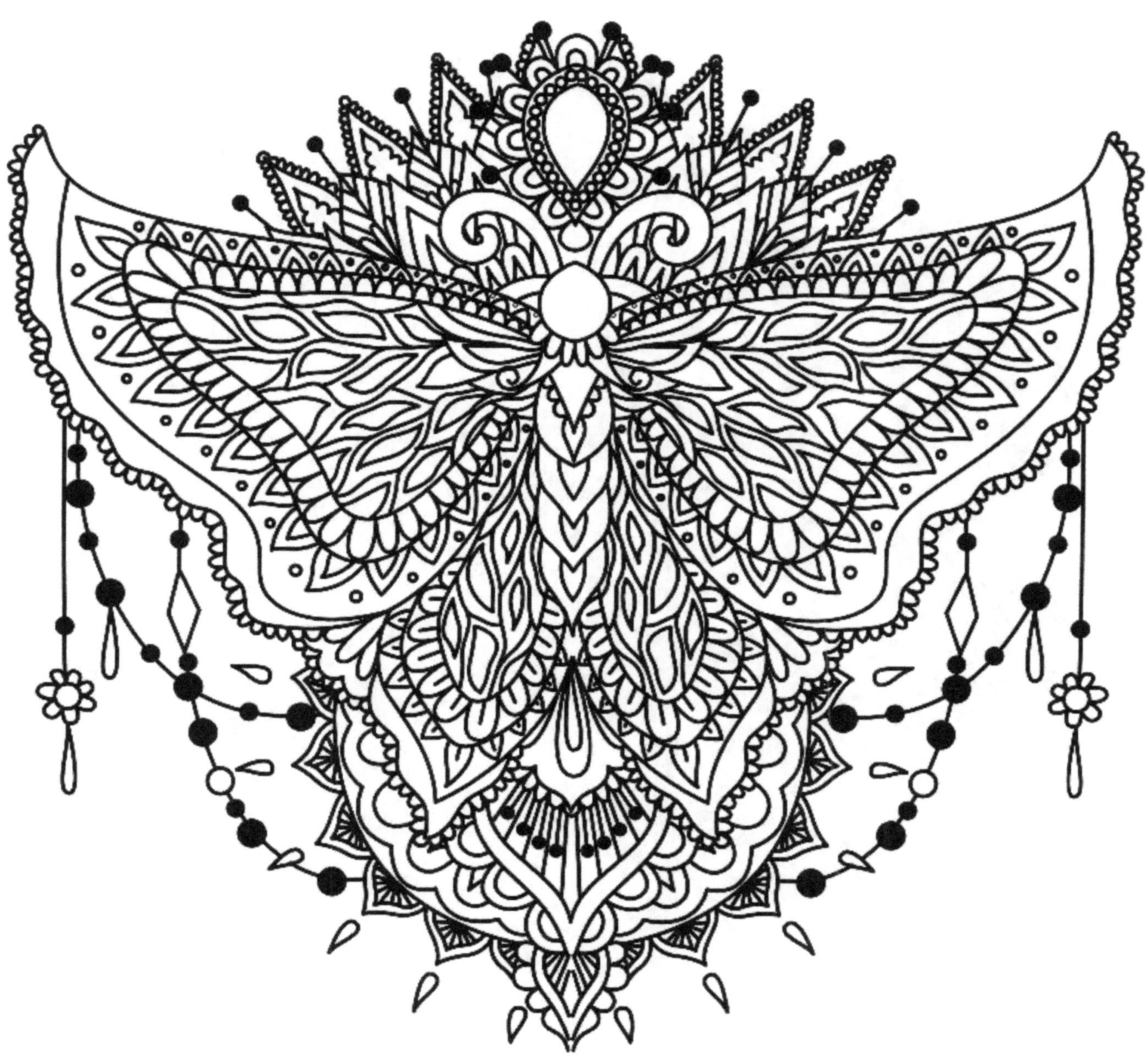

Think about how awesome it is that you're quitting smoking and getting healthy. If you start to weaken, remember your goal. Remember that quitting is a learning process. Be patient with yourself.

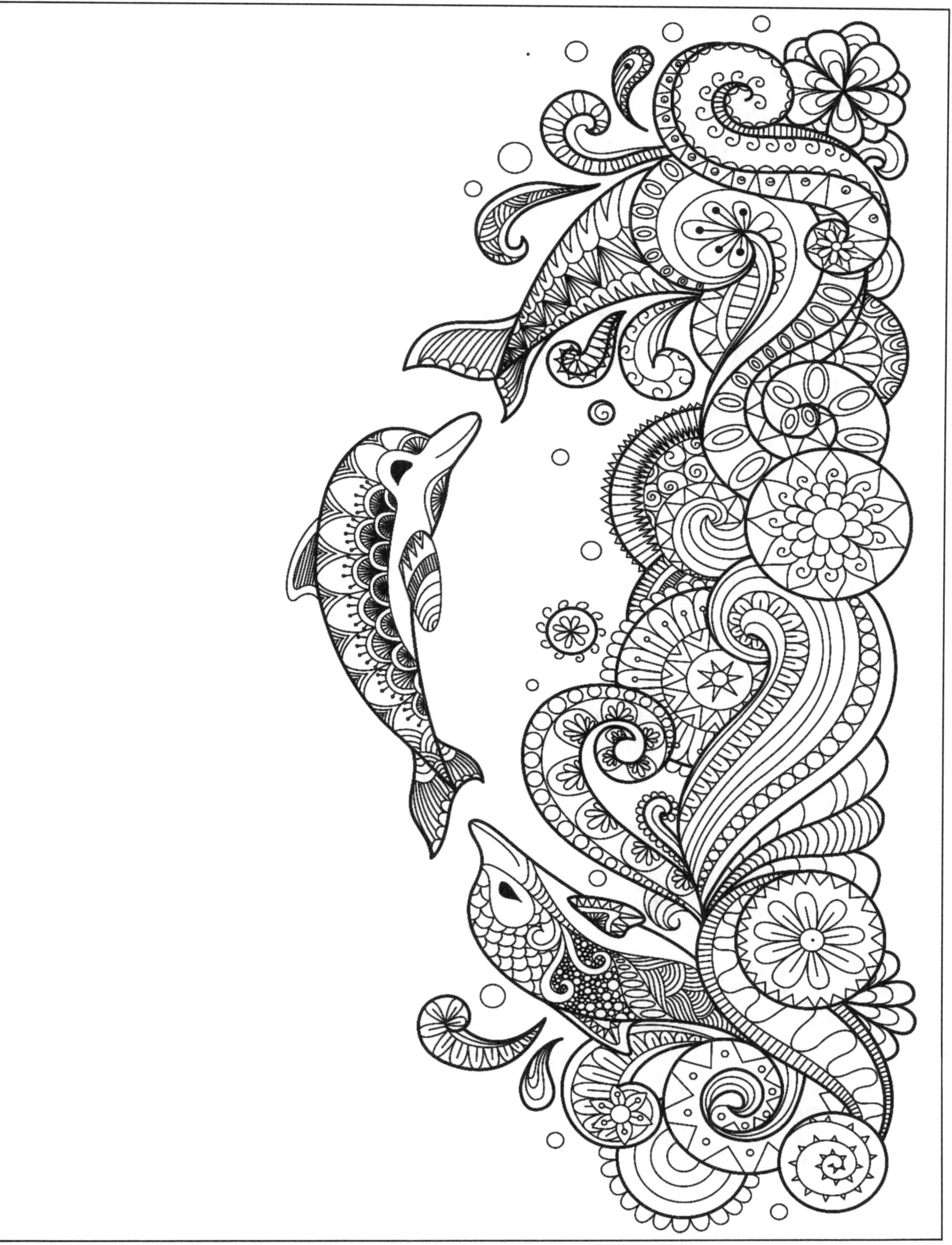

Kick the habit month 6

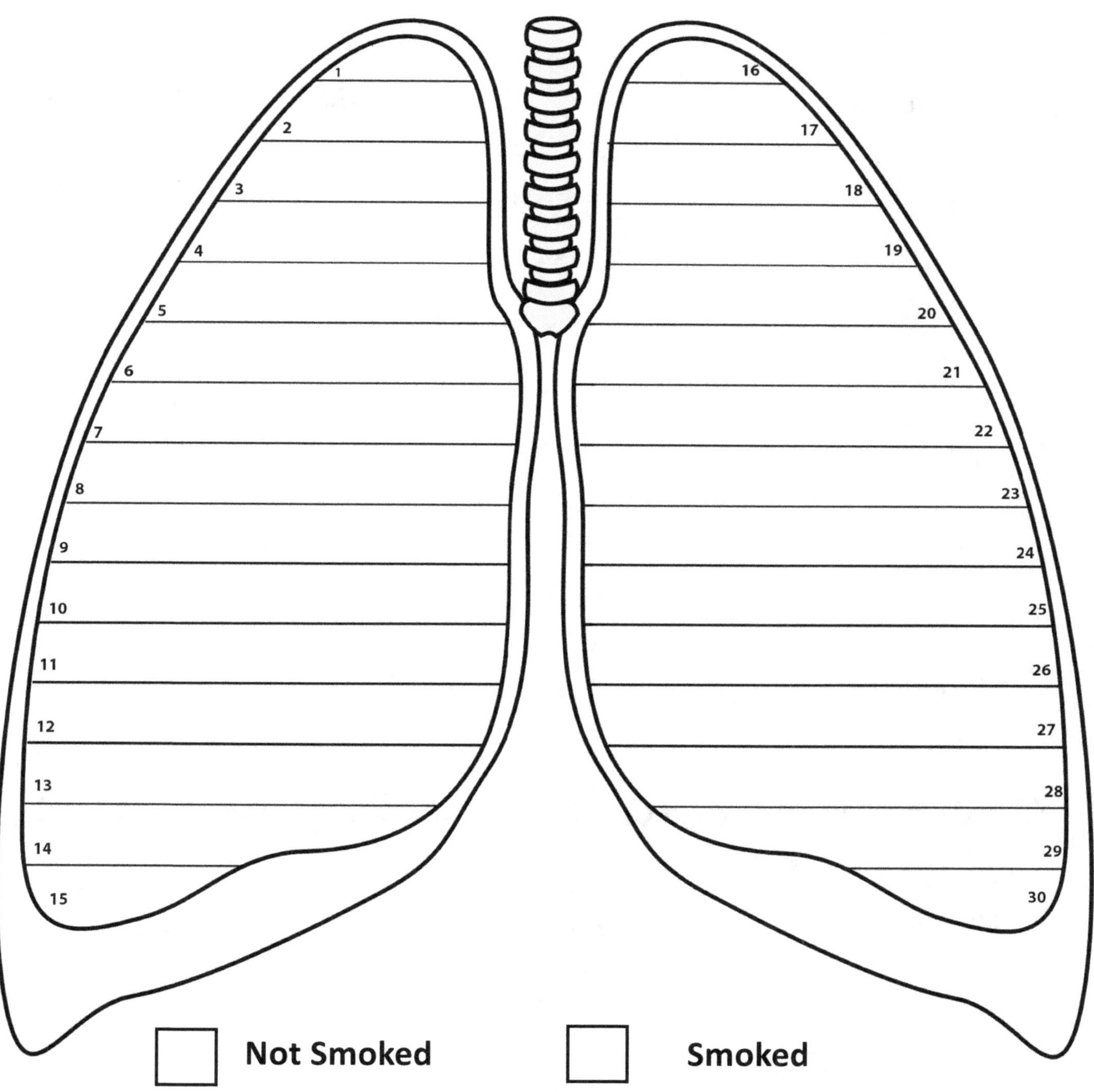

"You are greater than your addiction." - Nasia Davos

Week

MONTH:

WEEK:

WEEKLY WINS	WORK IN PROGRESS

One Step at a time, One Day at a time

MY GOALS	FAMILY GOALS	CAREER GOALS

Today

DAILY
PLANNER

MON

TUE

WED

THU

Today

FRI

SAT

SUN

enjoy your life

Week

MONTH:

WEEK:

WEEKLY WINS	WORK IN PROGRESS

One Step at a time, One Day at a time

MY GOALS	FAMILY GOALS	CAREER GOALS

Today

MON

TUE

WED

THU

Today

FRI

SAT

SUN

enjoy
your
life

Week

MONTH: WEEK:

WEEKLY WINS	WORK IN PROGRESS

One Step at a time, One Day at a time

MY GOALS	FAMILY GOALS	CAREER GOALS

Today

MON

TUE

WED

THU

Today

FRI

SAT

SUN

enjoy
your
life

Week

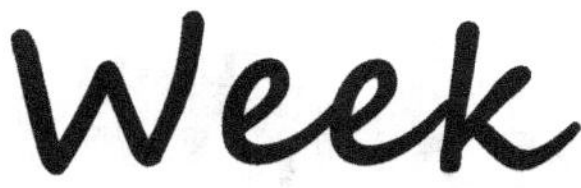

MONTH: **WEEK:**

WEEKLY WINS	WORK IN PROGRESS

One Step at a time, One Day at a time

MY GOALS	FAMILY GOALS	CAREER GOALS

Today

MON

TUE

WED

THU

Today

FRI

SAT

SUN

enjoy
your
life

Week

MONTH:

WEEK:

WEEKLY WINS

WORK IN PROGRESS

One Step at a time, One Day at a time

MY GOALS

FAMILY GOALS

CAREER GOALS

Today

MON

TUE

WED

THU

Today

FRI

SAT

SUN

enjoy your life

How I Felt

____

____

____

____

Combat Techniques

____

____

____

____

Reflections of this month

Color the stress away...

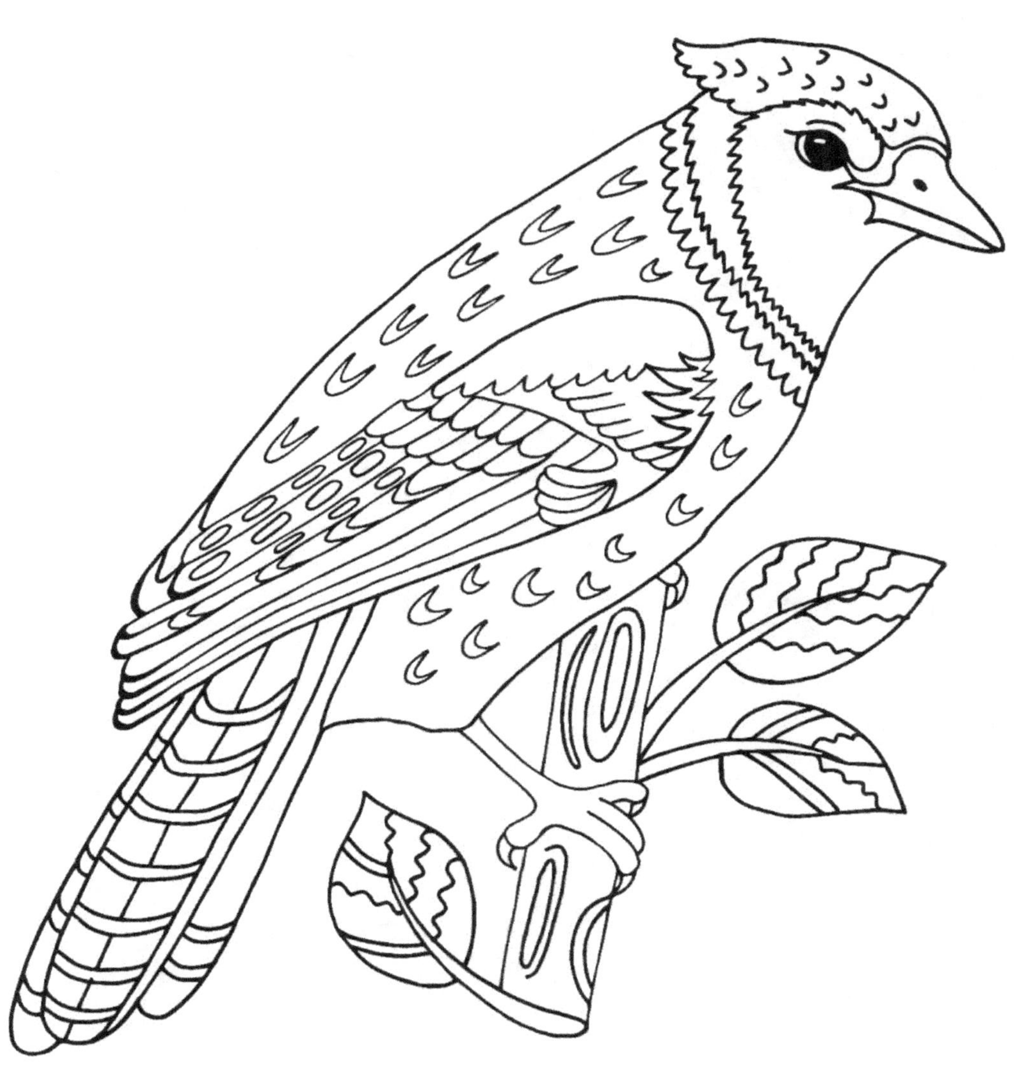

Create new habits and a non-smoking environment around you.

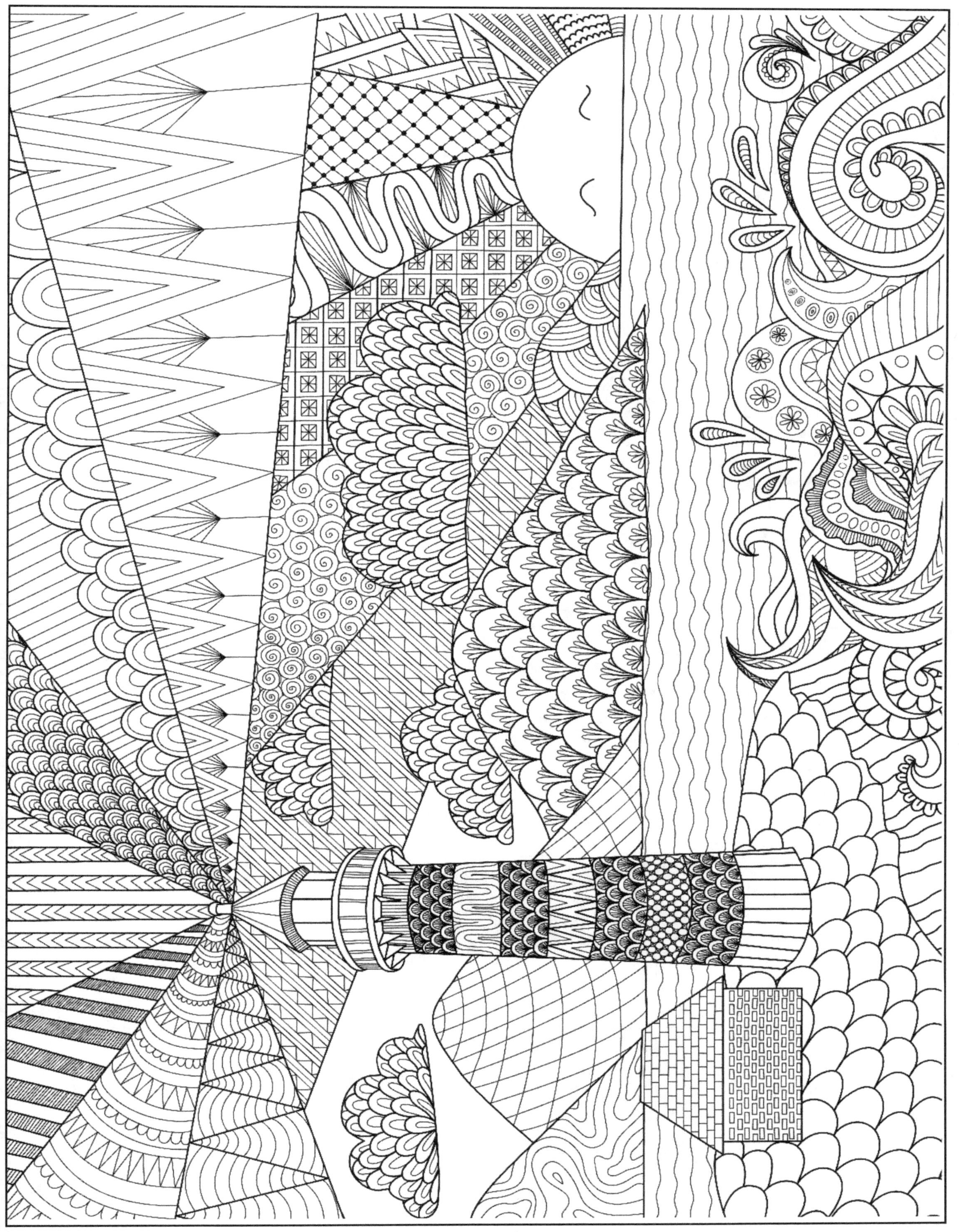

YOU DID IT!!
NOW KEEP IT UP!

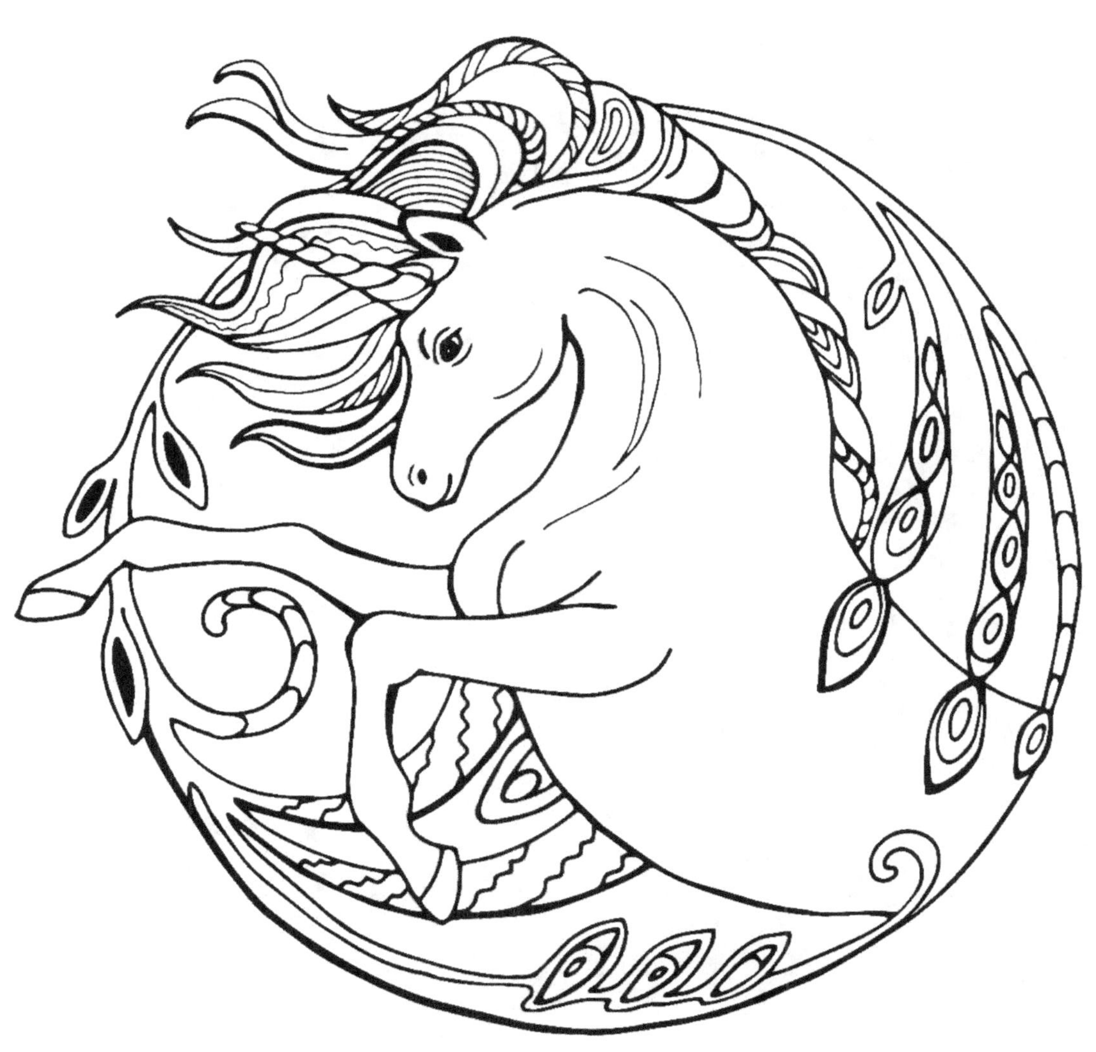

www.ingramcontent.com/pod-product-compliance
Lightning Source LLC
Chambersburg PA
CBHW081616250726
48657CB00009B/2591